Heaven's Health Service

A Reformation in Healthcare

Revised Edition

by

Vernon C. Sparks, M.D.

I0447262

Copyright © 1993, 2002, 2009, 2012

by
Vernon Sparks

Published
by

DIGITAL INSPIRATION
1481 Reagan Valley Road
Tellico Plains, TN 37385
www.vsdigitalinspiration.com

Contents

The Problem: A Healthcare Crisis

The Solution: Heaven's Plan

The Role and Response of Christ's Followers

Part I

The Problem:
A Healthcare Crisis

The Ills of Mankind

Heaven is all health. *Counsels on Health*, 28.

VERY few of us need to be reminded that we are living in a world plagued by disease and suffering. The total weight of human pain is immeasurable. Those of us fortunate enough to live in one of the developed countries have access to the most advanced and the most technical systems for the detection and the combating of disease ever known in the history of mankind. But in spite of the great efforts expended and the near miraculous breakthroughs in the field of modern medicine, millions worldwide still face lifetimes of far from ideal health. Each year one million persons in the world die from malaria. Each year three quarters of a million Americans die prematurely from hardening of the arteries and another one-half million from cancer. It is estimated that in 1989, 35,000 persons died from starvation worldwide for each day of the year. That number was equivalent to 100 fully loaded Jumbo Jets crashing every day for one year. These are only a few of the many health problems presently afflicting mankind. The following quotation is a marked understatement.

> Thousands of poor mortals with deformed, sickly bodies, shattered nerves, and gloomy minds, are dragging out a miserable existence. *Counsels on Health*, 18.

THE MODERN, scientific approach to the problem of disease has been based on the concept that for every disease problem there is a discoverable and treatable cause or causes. This rational approach to problems in the natural world has yielded remarkable, and at times nearly unbelievable, results. Almost daily we are made aware of new information regarding the cause of, or the cure for, some disease. Millions and even billions of dollars have been and are being spent for research in a noble attempt by mankind to alleviate the burden of illness. We are all aware of how epidemiology, sanitation and vaccinations have nearly eradicated a number of serious and sometimes devastating diseases such as polio, diphtheria, and the bubonic plague. It appears that smallpox as a disease-causing agent has been eradicated from this earth. However, in spite of the remarkable progress made in the fields of disease prevention, control and cure, suffering and ill health continue almost unabated. In 1971 America declared a "war on cancer." Billions of dollars have since been spent trying to learn better prevention and earlier diagnosis of, and improved treatment for, the many varieties of cancer. There has been remarkable progress with some varieties of cancer, but others have actually become more unyielding. The statistics on overall incidence of and death from cancer has improved very little, if any.

IT ALSO seems that when one disease appears to be conquered a new and even worse one takes its place. We are all very much aware of the current problem of AIDS. In the 1970s this new disease spread around the world essentially undetected, much to the embarrassment of the scientific community. Although much has been learned in the last few years about this lethal disorder, the twelve to thirteen million people worldwide estimated to already be infected with the AIDS virus, are presently given very little hope of escaping an untimely death.

COSTLY research continues seeking the etiology, or causes, of other diseases. New and more advanced techniques for treating these causes are being searched for and developed. Discoveries are being made faster than they can be distributed and applied. An increasing number of health personnel and facilities are unable to dispense modern medicine adequately even in the developed countries. In addition, copious research and development have resulted in an alarming increase in the cost of healthcare. In 1992 it cost Americans approximately 800 billion dollars for healthcare. United States healthcare leaders along with politicians, are appalled at the task of equally distributing modern health services. When one considers the financial costs of making modern healthcare available to all who need it on a worldwide basis the task is indeed staggering. For a number of years now there have been open and frank discussions of a "health crisis."

THESE problems are so immense that all possible solutions are being evaluated. New types of health workers are being trained. As mentioned, concentrated programs of research are being carried on in attempts to discover the causes of the various diseases. In addition, methods for caring for patients at home are being developed to help keep down expenses. New methods of distributing healthcare are being devised. New emphasis is being placed on preventive medicine with the goal of preventing the first inroads of disease. There is even an attempt to associate religion more closely with medical care as an important emotional and psychological aid in the patient's fight against disease.

ALONG with a worldwide deficit in healthcare workers, facilities and funds, several other very frustrating problems exist. One of these is the tendency of health personnel to congregate where living and working are the most convenient and comfortable rather than where their services are most needed. Another problem is that in many places the health profession is viewed the same way as other professions. It is considered to be part of the free enterprise system. Thus its fees and salaries usually are determined by the "law of supply and demand." Indeed, some aspects of healthcare are considered in many areas as big business. Another distressing problem is that of lack of interest on the part of many people regarding discoveries in the field of prevention. Related to this problem is the seeming inability of many persons to make permanent needed changes in their habits of living.

AS THEY study these multifaceted problems related to the disease and suffering pervading our present world, many people wonder if indeed there are answers. They recognize that conventional approaches are not working. They realize there must be a serious reevaluation of the old methods and a strengthening of their useful parts; however, many believe that any real hope for successfully conquering world health problems lies in newer methods and approaches. They see a tremendous need for a reformation in healthcare. Let us study deeper into the problems of disease and suffering and discover what form this reformation in healthcare must take if it is to meet with success.

The Source of the Solutions

IT IS ONLY logical to conclude that if the true cause or causes of disease can be discovered and removed, then success must be ours. In order to solve the problem of illness better than have our predecessors, we must know more than they have known. We must know who man is and where he came from. We must know what man was like before he became affected by disease. We must know more than we do about disease. We must discern what it is and where it came or comes from. If we can do these things then the solutions to our problems may not be as difficult or as far removed as they have appeared.

THOSE who believe in evolution as the origin of the human race seem to be having great difficulties in developing a truly effective healthcare system. In contrast, those who accept by faith the Bible's account of man's creation by an all-loving, all-powerful, Divine Being should find the problem much less difficult. Why? Because an effective healthcare system will be much easier to develop and implement if it follows the outline given for it by mankind's Creator.

BEFORE advancing further, let us state firmly that all who are sincerely concerned about the problems related to disease and pain cannot be halfhearted in their desire for real answers and permanent solutions. Symptomatic, palliative healthcare is not their ideal, and is ethically permissible only until a true solution is found. Once a true solution is discovered all healthcare workers should apply the new, effective treatment. Those who do not implement the most effective methods available do not have the best interests of their patients at heart and should be considered guilty of malpractice.

Who Man Is

THE CREATION of man was the crowning act of the Creator. Being created in God's image, man was created to glorify God.

Man was the crowning act of the creation of God, made in the image of God, and designed to be a counterpart of God. *Temperance*, 11.

Above all lower orders of being, God designed that man, the crowning work of His creation, should express His thought and reveal His glory. *Testimonies for the Church*, Vol. 8, 264.

Natural Law

SCIENCE has discovered that the natural world operates harmoniously by obedience to definite rules or laws. Only by strict observance of these laws can man succeed in endeavors such as space travel and electronic communications. In the care and cure of the human body man can also succeed only by following natural laws.

When God had made man in His image, the human form was perfect in all its arrangements, but it was without life. Then a personal, self existing God breathed into that form the breath of life, and man became a living, breathing, intelligent being. All parts of the human organism were put in action. The heart, the arteries, the veins, the tongue, the hands, the feet, the senses, the perceptions of the mind,—all began their work, and all were placed under law. Ibid.

DISOBEDIENCE to these laws results in disease and diminished body function.

For every offense committed against the laws of health the transgressor must pay the penalty in his own body. *Counsels on Health*, 595.

MAN WAS originally created with vigorous vital force and with a reason and willpower in charge of the body and its impulses. He was capable of obeying the natural laws of his being and was thus assured of health. In addition, he was given access to the tree of life which contained properties providing continued life.

> They [newly created Adam and Eve] were full of the vigor imparted by the tree of life, and their intellectual power was but little less than that of the angels. . . . In order to possess an endless existence, man must continue to partake of the tree of life. Deprived of this, his vitality would gradually diminish until life should become extinct. *Patriarchs and Prophets*, 50, 60.

Disobedience

DISEASE and suffering and death were unknown before man disobeyed God's natural and spiritual laws. Even then the results were not fully felt for many years.

> Man came from the hand of God perfect in every faculty of mind and body; in perfect soundness, therefore in perfect health. It took more then two thousand years of indulgence of appetite and lustful passions to create such a state of things in the human organism as would lessen vital force. Through successive generations the tendency was more swiftly downward. Indulgence of appetite and passion combined led to excess and violence; debauchery and abominations of every kind weakened the energies, and brought upon the race diseases of every type, until the vigor and glory of the first generations passed away, and in the third generation from Adam, man began to show signs of decay. *Testimonies for the Church*, vol. 4, 29.

THROUGH disobedience man lost his kingly control over the impulses of his body. He lost access to the tree of life. He no longer, of himself, could obey the natural laws of his being. Today man suffers from disharmony in his being due to his own disobedience, and also to his inherited tendencies and weaknesses toward disease passed on by the disobedient generations before him.

A Devil to Fight

MAN, HOWEVER, is not solely responsible for his disobedience to natural law. To know the cause of disease one must know of Satan. The devil, who was the instigator of disobedience to natural law and who is continuously active in propagating the resultant problems. Anyone working toward obedience to all natural law has the devil to fight, and any designed program to truly overcome disease must include means to overcome him.

> It is Satan's determined work to destroy the image of God in man. *General Conference Daily Bulletin*, March 2, 1897 (*Story of Our Health Message*, 289).

> Satan is the originator of disease; and the physician is warring against his work and power. *Testimonies for the Church*, vol. 5, 443–444.

The Problem of Sin

MAN WAS created a living soul made up of physical, mental and moral natures or powers. See *Education*, 210. Our mental powers are our ability to reason and to make decisions. Our moral powers are our inherent need for and ability to form social relationships with other intelligent beings including God Himself. What affects one aspect of man affects all of man. To effectively combat disease, one must understand well the wholistic relationship within man. The importance of this truth is well illustrated by the fact that ninety percent of disease has its foundation in the mind or mental powers and that many are suffering more from problems related to social and spiritual needs than they are of problems related to physical needs.

> Sickness of the mind [mental powers] prevails everywhere. Nine-tenths of the diseases from which men suffer have their foundation here. Ibid., 444.

> Many are suffering from maladies of the soul [moral pow-

ers] far more than from diseases of the body, and they will find
no relief until they shall come to Christ, the well-spring of life.
Complaints of weariness, loneliness, and dissatisfaction, will then
cease. Satisfying joys will give vigor to the mind, and health
and vital energy to the body. The burden of sin, with its unrest
and unsatisfied desires, lies at the very foundation of a large
share of the maladies the sinner suffers. Ibid., vol. 4, 579.

FROM THESE statements we can conclude that any serious attempt to cure man's suffering and disease must include means for
healing the diseases of the mind and soul as well as of the body. Thus
we see that the disease problem is much bigger than most people
realize. This fact explains such persons' inability to cope with disease and for society in general to be unable to develop healthcare
systems that truly solve the broad problems of ill health. Any cure
has to be more powerful than the problem it is intended to alleviate.
A healthcare system, to be effective, must include not only a cure for
the physical ills of man but also for the sicknesses and deficiencies
of man's mental and moral natures and thus for sin itself.

Part II

The Solution: Heaven's Plan

Knowledge Essential to Success

TO EFFECTIVELY treat man and his diseases we must first know the laws—natural and spiritual—which control the harmonious interrelationships between man's physical, mental and moral selves. Obedience to these laws will not only prevent disease but in the majority of the cases it will also prove effective in eradicating disease and restoring health. Any narrower approach to the human disease problem will finally prove to be too limited and only palliative rather than curative.

> My people are destroyed for lack of knowledge. Hosea 4:6.

BEFORE sin entered, man was aware of the laws that reigned in his being. With generations of disobedience and disease, this knowledge was lost. Many of the laws of health (primarily those of diet, hygiene and sanitation) were again revealed to the Israelites at Mount Sinai, along with the spiritual laws governing the spiritual health of man. It was God's purpose that these laws of the body, mind and soul should be practiced by the Israelites and by them be promulgated throughout the world. Thus God was attempting at that time to solve man's disease problem.

WE KNOW this attempt by God failed because the Israelites failed to do their part. Many of these laws were again lost sight of as evidenced by the history of the Dark Ages. During these centuries of ignorance, millions suffered and died within sight of monasteries where Bibles containing the principles of disease prevention were stored away, unstudied, thus preventing light from shining upon the people.

AT PRESENT, we are said to be living in a period of enlightenment. As previously noted, it is true that some progress toward the alleviation of suffering has been made. Some causes of disease have been discovered and the prevalence of some diseases has been markedly reduced. A few diseases have even been eradicated. This progress, however, has required the strenuous efforts of thousands of researchers over many years; and it has required the expenditure of billions of dollars. We have to admit that at least some of this effort and expense was essential and that it brought results perhaps not obtainable in any other way, considering man's sin problem. One must wonder, however, how much of this same progress could have been accomplished, and the intense labor and great expense made unnecessary, if mankind had accepted and practiced by faith the laws of health as revealed in the Bible. This wondering is even greater if one is aware that God has revealed to His people in a body of writing called the Spirit of Prophecy these laws of health in an amplified form.

Health Reform

GOD HAS again, out of His great love and compassion, made known to man the laws which govern his body. These have been given again to mankind in association with the laws that govern his mind and his spiritual health. The knowledge of and practice of these innate laws of our beings have been referred to as Health Reform. This knowledge and practice are a vital part of the only Health Plan comprehensive enough to have any chance of truly solving the problem of disease. Health Reform is not of any man's devising; it is of God. It is not earthly, but divine.

> It is a great thing to insure health by placing ourselves in right relations to the laws of life. *Counsels on Health*, 49.

IT IS ONLY reasonable to believe that man can preserve health, and can prevent and cure most diseases by obedience to the laws governing his being. It is also only sensible to believe that no one would have a better knowledge of these laws than the Manufacturer or Creator of mankind. It is also only logical for a loving God to make these laws known once again to us as we near the climax of His work of restoring the body, mind, and soul of man to the position he was originally designed to fill.

> God does not require His children to deny themselves to the injury of physical strength. He requires them to obey natural law, to preserve physical health. Nature's path is the road He makes out and it is broad enough for any Christian. Ibid., 74.

> My son, attend to my words; incline thine ear unto my sayings. Let them not depart from thine eyes; keep them in the midst of thine heart. For they are life unto those that find them, and health to all their flesh. Proverbs 4:20–22.

THE PRINCIPLES of health as outlined in the Bible and amplified by the writings of Mrs. E. G. White are indeed broad. They cover all aspects of our living habits and surroundings. It is amazing how much detail they present.

Three Main Purposes

THERE are three main and progressive purposes of Health Reform. The first is that of lessening suffering.

> The work of health reform is the Lord's means for lessening suffering in our world. *Testimonies for the Church*, vol. 9, 112.

ONCE SUFFERING is relieved, health reform's second purpose, that of opening doors to other truths, is frequently realized.

> I have been informed by my guide that not only should those who believe the truth practice health reform, but they should also teach it diligently to others; for it will be an agency through which the truth can be presented to the attention of unbelievers. They will reason that if we have such sound ideas in regard to health and temperance, there must be something in our religious belief that is worth investigation. If we backslide in health reform we shall lose much of our influence with the outside world. *Evangelism*, 514.

HEALTH reform's third main purpose is to aid in spiritual growth. Adoption of the principles of health assists in, and is also an essential part of, spiritual perfection.

> When they break away from all health-destroying indulgence, they will have a clearer perception of what constitutes true godliness. A wonderful change will be seen in the religious experience. *Counsels on Health*, 579.

> God demands that the appetites be cleansed, and that self-denial be practiced in regard to those things which are not good. This is a work that will have to be done before His people can stand before Him a perfected people. *Testimonies for the Church*, vol. 9, 153–154.

Anatomy and Physiology

MANY MIGHT ask, "But how can the principles of health reform be effectively applied to the lives of man?" First, man must have an intelligent understanding of the anatomy and physiology of his own being.

> From the first dawn of reason, the human mind should become intelligent in regard to the physical structure. Here Jehovah has given a specimen of Himself; for man was made in the image of God. *Medical Ministry*, 221.

> They [parents] should be practical physiologists that they may know what are and what are not correct physical habits. *Counsels on Health*, 39.

Knowledge That Motivates

KNOWLEDGE of what one should do however is not enough. Man must also have the will power to practice that which he knows. Knowledge of the well-proven relationship between smok-

ing and cancer has not been very effective in eradicating the to-
bacco-smoking habit because many smokers lack sufficient power
to cease smoking. Only God's health plan provides for such deficiencies.

MAN'S MOTIVATION to better his habits of living is greatly
strengthened when he understands that his body is a temple of
the Holy Ghost, that it really belongs to God, that it has only
been entrusted to him, and that his eternal destiny is affected by
how he cares for it. Motivation is also increased by knowing that
God's laws of health are just as sacred as God's Ten Command-
ment law and that obedience to both is enjoined by God's last
message to mankind.

> The physical penalty of disregarding the laws of nature will
> appear in the form of sickness, ruined constitutions and even
> death itself. But a settlement is also to be made by and by, with
> God. *Temperance*, 143.

> It is just as much sin to violate the laws of our being as to
> break one of the Ten Commandments, for we cannot do either
> without breaking God's law. *Testimonies for the Church*, vol. 2,
> 70–71.

> We are not our own. We have been purchased with a dear
> price, even the sufferings and death of the Son of God. If we
> could understand this, and fully realize it, we would feel a great
> responsibility resting upon us to keep ourselves in the very
> best condition of health, that we might render to God perfect
> service. Ibid., 354.

> The knowledge that man is to be a temple for God, a habi-
> tation for the revealing of His glory, should be the highest
> incentive to the care and development of our physical pow-
> ers. *The Ministry of Healing*, 271.

> To make plain natural law, and urge the obedience of it, is
> the work that accompanies the third angel's message, to prepare
> a people for the coming of the Lord. *Testimonies for the Church*,
> vol. 3, 161.

THE NATURAL laws of our being are an essential and integral part of the three angels' messages, the last warning messages given to our world, found in Revelation 14. This fact can better be understood when one realizes that the three angels' messages enjoin obedience to God's laws. This obedience includes both the laws of God in the natural world and His laws in the spiritual world. Those who make these laws plain to the world and teach the moral obligation to obey them are called repairers of the breech.

> And they that shall be of thee shall build the old waste places; thou shalt raise up the foundations of many generations; and thou shalt be called, The repairer of the breach, The restorer of paths to dwell in. Isaiah 58:12.

ELDER J. H. Waggoner, in referring to the general principles of health reform, made the following statement:

> As mere physiological and hygienic truths, they might be studied by some at their leisure and by others laid aside as of little consequence; but when placed on a level with the great truths of the third angel's message by the sanction and authority of God's Spirit, and so declared to be the means whereby a weak people may be made strong to overcome, and our diseased bodies cleansed and fitted for translation, then it comes to us as an essential part of present truth to be received with the blessing of God, or rejected at our peril. *The Story of Our Health Message*, 79–80.

HEALTH reform is destined to play an increasingly important role in the final message to a world lost in physical and spiritual sin.

> When the third angel's message is received in its fullness, health reform will be given its place in the councils of the Conference, in the work of the church, in the home, at the table, and in all the household arrangements. Then the right arm will serve and protect the body. *Testimonies for the Church*, vol. 6, 327.

Will Power That Is Effective

ONE OF the frequent problems encountered in the field of health is the lack of power to put into practice that which one knows is right. Man, through sin, has lost his kingly control of reason ruling the impulses of the body. Man, of himself, can no more obey fully the laws of God in his physical life than he can obey fully the laws of God in his spiritual life. Righteousness by faith in Jesus Christ is just as necessary for success in the field of health as it is for success in the spiritual realm.

> Apart from divine power, no genuine reform can be effected. Human barriers against natural and cultivated tendencies are but as the sandbank against the torrent. Not until the life of Christ becomes a vitalizing power in our lives can we resist the temptations that assail us from within and from without. *The Ministry of Healing*, 130.

> Through the right exercise of the will, an entire change may be made in the life. By yielding up the will to Christ, we ally ourselves with divine power. We receive strength from above to hold us steadfast. A pure and noble life, a life of victory over appetite and lust, is possible to everyone who will unite his weak, wavering human will to the omnipotent, unwavering will of God. Ibid., 176.

DIVINE power which is available to man is the secret of success in Heaven's Health Service.

Readily Available Remedies

OBEDIENCE to the laws of health is essential in the preservation of health and the prevention of disease. Obedience to these same laws is also a great therapeutic aid in combating disease and thus in recovering health. In addition to giving us Health Reform—obedience to natural law—as a therapeutic aid, Heaven has also made available important natural remedies.

Pure air, sunlight, abstemiousness, rest, exercise, proper diet, the use of water, trust in divine power—these are the true remedies. Ibid., 127.

Teach nurses and patients the value of those health-restoring agencies that are freely provided by God, and the usefulness of simple things that are easily obtained. . . .

Always study and teach the use of the simplest remedies, and the special blessing of the Lord may be expected to follow the use of these means which are within the reach of the common people. *Selected Messages*, book 2, 298–299.

The Source of Healing

THE STUDY of remedies brings us to the matter of what is the source of healing. We have recovered health so many times after visiting the doctor and taking medication, or after using simple home remedies, that we tend to believe that the source of healing is found in the treatment. However, man and his modern technology or simple remedies can only help remove the causes of disease and aid recovery; the actual healing and restoring power comes from God through nature.

Whenever man accomplishes anything, whether in spiritual or in temporal lines, he should bear in mind that he does it through cooperation with his Maker. There is great necessity for us to realize our dependence on God. *Christ's Object Lessons*, 82.

Let physicians teach the people that restorative power is not in drugs, but in nature. *Counsels on Health*, 90.

Through the agencies of nature, God is working, day by day, hour by hour, moment by moment, to keep us alive, to build up and restore us. When any part of the body sustains injury, a healing process is at work to restore soundness. But the power working through these agencies is the power of God. All life-giving power is from Him. When one recovers from disease, it is God who restores him. Ibid., 168.

THUS THOSE who are desirous of developing an effective healthcare program must understand well how to bring suffering humanity into as close a harmony as possible with nature and with nature's God—the source of healing.

Remedy Relationships

BEFORE progressing further, let us attempt to clarify the relation between health reform, nature's remedies, and modern therapeutics. In this area extremism readily develops. There are these who believe that nature's remedies, combined with trust in divine power, are all that is needed to heal every manner of illness. By some purported health reformers all modern rational therapeutics are considered by these persons to be unnecessary and perhaps even evil as if from the devil. This belief is one form of extremism. Many others have noted the remarkable improvements in health brought about by modern therapeutics apparently without regard to Health Reform or nature's remedies, and they tend to believe the latter two modalities are outdated and thus of little importance. This tendency is another form of extremism. Both approaches to healthcare will be found, in the long run, to be false.

> God has permitted a flood of light to be poured upon the world in discoveries in science. *Signs of the Times*, March 13, 1884.

IT APPEARS that in these last days a loving God has permitted man to discover many of His laws governing the health and diseases of the human body. By snatching man back from the brink of the grave modern therapeutics serve many times to give wayward man another opportunity to get acquainted with his Creator and to accept Him as his Saviour.

IN THE realm of spiritual health, revelations of its governing principles are given to man in an additive form. Thus newer truth does not negate previous truth, but is to be used to add to or to build upon the old. This principle is also true in the realm of physical health.

The principles of health reform and the use of nature's true remedies are always to be utilized, while modern rational therapeutics are to be resorted to only as necessary. The newer truth is not to replace the older truth nor the complex concept the simpler one, but they are to be added on as needed.

OBEDIENCE to nature's laws (Health Reform), the wise use of nature's remedies, and the use as needed of modern therapeutics all have an "essential" part to play in Heaven's Health Service and should usually be resorted to in that order. First and most important is the role of Health Reform in building up and maintaining optimal health. If disease does get hold, these same principles, in conjunction with nature's true remedies, will be effective in the majority of cases in ridding the body of disease and thus preparing the way for nature's restorative power. However, this side of eternity, there will always be those who need the aid of many of modern medicine's rational therapeutics.

MOST WILL recognize the need for, and the benefit of, modern diagnostics, vaccinations and surgery. Disobedience to the laws of health can also create a need for modern medications.

> Ill health in a variety of forms, if effect could be traced to the cause, would reveal the sure result of flesh eating. The disuse of meats, with healthful dishes nicely prepared to take the place of flesh meats, would place a large number of the sick and suffering ones in a fair way of recovering their health, without the use of drugs. But if the physician encourages a meat-eating diet to his invalid patients, then he will make a necessity for the use of drugs. *Medical Ministry*, 222.

AS WE ARE all aware, the majority of modern therapeutic agents can have certain undesirable and sometimes dangerous side-effects. Thus their use should be controlled by a well-trained physician, and they should be used only when the dangers of the potential side-effects of the therapeutic agent are outweighed by the potential and impending adverse effects of the disease. The principle of choosing the lesser of two evils should be followed.

W E SEE the application of this principle in the cases of individuals who have gran mal seizures. These individuals suffer the risk of some permanent brain injury with each seizure. This is in addition to the danger of potential injury from falling or striking objects during a seizure. It is nearly impossible to prevent these seizures by the simple remedies of diet, exercise, herbs and so forth. Those who prevent the seizures by taking medication on a regular basis under the supervision of a physician tend to have less health problems from the medications than they would from the seizures if they did not prevent them with the medication. The lesser of the two evils is usually putting up with the side effects of the medication rather than suffering the more serious consequences of seizures without the medication.

T HUS GOD'S Health Service has three divinely provided bulwarks against disease and suffering. The first one, obedience to natural law, along with utilization of the tree of life, will be used throughout eternity to maintain and strengthen health. At Christ's second coming, when these corruptible, mortal bodies are changed into incorruptible, immortal flesh, modern rational therapeutics as well as the simple natural remedies will no longer be needed in God's universe.

A Wholistic Work

G OD NOT only has His fortifications against disease, He also has His way of providing them to suffering humanity. His method of distributing healthcare is called medical missionary work, and He sent His Son to this earth to give us a practical demonstration of how it is to be done. Jesus' example raised the profession of healthcare to levels never before witnessed and seldom since patterned after. He combined healthcare and spiritual care into one profession. Thus He was able to treat the whole man, providing mankind the opportunity for both eternal health and eternal life. He raised the health profession from a level of commercialism and placed it on its true level as a self sacrificing, high, holy, and sacred mission.

Healthcare was placed on an equal basis with the ministry. In fact, it was made an essential part of the gospel ministry.

> Christ was bound up in all branches of the work of God. He made no division. He did not feel that He was infringing on the work of the physician when He healed the sick. *Testimonies for the Church*, vol. 6, 242.

> Our work is clearly defined. As the Father sent His only begotten Son into our world, even so Christ sends us, His disciples, as His medical missionary workers. In fulfilling this high and holy mission, we are to do the will of God. *Medical Ministry*, 24.

CHRIST came to this earth to provide healing and salvation to the whole man and He has ordained that the medical missionary work is to go forward hand in hand with the ministry. The work for the body and the work for the soul are not to be separated.

> If the work of the third angel's message is carried on in the right lines, the ministry will not be given an inferior place, nor will the poor and sick be neglected. In His word God has united these two lines of work and no man should divorce them. *Counsels on Health*, 515.

> Medical missionary work is in no case to be divorced from the gospel ministry. The Lord has specified that the two shall be as closely connected as the arm is with the body. Without this union neither part of the work is complete. The medical missionary work is the gospel in illustration. *Testimonies for the Church*, vol. 6, 240–241.

THE WORK place of the medical missionary is a broad field. It encompasses the alleviation of all physical, mental and spiritual suffering. It is best described in chapter fifty-eight of Isaiah.

> Is not this the fast that I have chosen? to loose the bands of wickedness, to undo the heavy burdens, and to let the oppressed go free, and that ye break every yoke? Is it not to deal thy bread to the hungry, and that thou bring the poor that are cast out to thy house? when thou seest the naked, that thou cover him; and that thou hide not thyself from thine own flesh? Isaiah 58:6–7.

I cannot too strongly urge all our church members, all who are true missionaries, all who believe the third angel's message, all who turn away their feet from the Sabbath, to consider the message of the fifty-eighth chapter of Isaiah. The work of beneficence enjoined in this chapter is the work that God requires His people to do at this time. *Testimonies for the Church*, vol. 6, 265.

But every effort to heal the imbalance brought about by sin is in reality part of genuine medical missionary work. Wilbur K. Nelson, and Leo R. VanDolson, *The Role of Religion in Health Education*, 1972, pp. 1–2, Loma Linda, Ca., School of Health, LLU.

THIS WORK for suffering humanity which Christ did and which He has enjoined and empowered His church to continue, will be seen by the world as a new, strange and distinct work.

The study of surgery and other medical science receives much attention in the world, but the true science of medical missionary work, carried forward as Christ carried it, is new and strange to the denominational churches and to the world. But it will find its rightful place when as a people who have had great light, Seventh-day Adventists awaken to their responsibilities and improve their opportunities. *Evangelism*, 518.

Self-denial and self-sacrifice are to be shown. We are to work as Christ worked, in simplicity and meekness, in lowliness and consecration. Thus we shall be enabled to do a work distinct from all other missionary work in our world. *Testimonies for the Church*, vol. 8, 183-184.

Heaven's Healthcare Workers

JUST AS the success of heaven's plan for suffering man calls for a type of work not normally done, just so it requires a different type and class of worker.

HISTORICALLY, until recent times, knowledge regarding health and the treatment of disease was held mainly by priests or other religious practitioners. These dual tasks were given by God to the priests of the health-progressive nation of Israel. This union of profession was also exemplified by Christ, the greatest medical missionary ever known.

> I know that an intimate relationship should ever exist between the medical missionary work and the gospel ministry. They are bound together in sacred union as one work, and are never to be divorced. *Counsels on Health*, 528.

THIS UNION entails more than cooperation between ministers and health workers, For anyone to be able to do the Lord's type of work for suffering humanity, he, individually, must be able to treat the soul as well as the body.

> In one hand they are to carry the gospel for the relief of sin-burdened souls; and in the other hand they are to carry remedies for the relief of physical suffering. Thus they will be true medical missionaries for God. *Medical Ministry*, 328.

THE HEALTH professionals and the spiritual professionals are to carry on this unified work. They are to be considered medical missionary evangelists.

> In this school many workers are to be qualified with the ability of physicians, to labor not in professional lines as physicians, but as medical missionary evangelists. Ibid., 58.

> The nurses who are trained in our institutions are to be fitted up to go out as medical missionary evangelists, uniting the ministry of the work with that of physical healing. *Testimonies for the Church*, vol. 9, 171.

> Let our ministers, who have gained an experience in preaching the word, learn to give simple treatments, and then labor intelligently as medical missionary evangelists. Ibid., 172.

THIS UNIFIED work is enjoined upon the physician.

> The Redeemer expects our physicians to make the saving of souls their first work. *Medical Ministry*, 37.

Every medical practitioner, whether he acknowledges it or not, is responsible for the souls as well as the bodies of his patients. The Lord expects of us much more than we often do for Him. Every physician should be a devoted, intelligent, gospel medical missionary, familiar with Heaven's remedy for the sin-sick soul as well as with the science of healing bodily disease. Ibid., 31.

This unified work is also enjoined upon the minister. Some utterly fail to realize the importance of missionaries being also medical missionaries. A gospel minister will be twice as successful in his work if he understands how to treat disease. Ibid., 245.

Ministers, do not confine your work to giving Bible instruction. Do practical work. Seek to restore the sick to health. This is true ministry. Remember that the restoration of the body prepares the way for restoration of the soul. Ibid., 240.

If our ministers would work earnestly to obtain an education in medical missionary lines they would be far better fitted to do the work Christ did as a medical missionary. By diligent study and practice, they can become so well acquainted with the principles of health reform that wherever they go they will be a great blessing to the people they meet. Ibid., 239.

TWO OF the less obvious benefits from this combination of labor are the following. It will help us avoid the tendency to heal just for the sake of temporal, palliative healing. By breaking down prejudice, it will also enable us to work longer where there are circumstances adverse to the preaching of the gospel.

Those who engage in this work should be consecrated to God, and not make it their only object to treat the body merely to cure disease, thus working from the popular physicians standpoint but to be spiritual fathers, to minister to diseased minds, and point sin-sick souls to the never failing remedy, the Saviour who died for them. *Testimonies for the Church*, vol. 3, 168.

I wish to tell you that soon there will be no work done in ministerial lines but medical missionary work. *Counsels on Health*, 533.

THUS MINISTERS and physicians are to do the same type of work. Each may give emphasis in the line for which he has the most specialized training, but the missionary physician's work is to so approximate the sacred work of the minister, that he too is to be ordained and authorized to baptize those whom he has won.

> The work of the true medical missionary is largely a spiritual work. It includes prayer and the laying on of hands; he therefore should be as sacredly set apart for his work as is the minister of the gospel. Those who are selected to act the part of missionary physicians are to be set apart as such. This will strengthen them against the temptations to withdraw from the sanitarium work to engage in private practice. No selfish motives should be allowed to draw the worker from his post of duty. Ibid., 540.

> The evangelist who is prepared to minister to a diseased body is given the grandest opportunity of ministering to the sin-sick soul. Such an evangelist should be empowered to administer baptism to those who are converted and desire baptism. *Evangelism*, 513.

GOD DOES not leave all of His healthcare to be done by professional missionary evangelists. He also asks literature evangelists to aid in this work. In fact, God enlists every member of His church in this grand labor for souls. Such a body of workers would be a tremendous aid in solving the problem of the constant shortage of health workers.

> It is medical missionaries that are needed all through the field. Canvassers should improve every opportunity granted them to learn how to treat disease. *Medical Ministry*, 249.

> We have come to a time when every member of the church should take hold of medical missionary work. . . . The members of the church are in need of an awakening, that they may realize their responsibility to impart these truths. *Testimonies for the Church*, vol. 7, 62.

> The members (of the church) are to be so established in the faith that they will have an intelligent knowledge of medical missionary work. They are to follow Christ's example, minister-

ing to those around them. *Medical Ministry*, 315

Our Sabbathkeeping families should keep their minds filled with helpful principles of health reform and other lines of truth, that they may be a help to their neighbors. Be practical missionaries. Gather up all the knowledge possible that will help to combat disease. This may be done by those who are diligent students. Ibid., 320.

Medical Missionary Training

WE MUST remember that medical missionary work (enjoined upon all church members) consists of treating both physical and spiritual disease. One may question as to where to obtain information regarding health and the treatment of disease from which God's health workers can learn to do successful work. We must recognize that God only is the source of true knowledge. Thus workers are to become educated along health lines as well as along spiritual lines by the study of God's Word and the Spirit of Prophecy. Other authors, in either of these fields, should be judged by the inspired counsel and only that information which is in harmony with inspired counsel should be utilized. Truth in the field of physical and spiritual health will not only be in harmony with and supportive of the Bible and the Spirit of Prophecy, but it will also be in harmony with a true understanding of the Creator's natural laws in the areas of anatomy, physiology, biochemistry and pathology.

The principles of health reform are found in the Word of God. *Medical Ministry*, 259.

God has permitted a flood of light to be poured upon the world in discoveries in science. *Signs of the Times*, March 13, 1884.

All can do something. Let our people show that they have a living interest in medical missionary work. Let them prepare themselves for usefulness by studying the books that have been written for our instruction in these lines. These books deserve much more attention and appreciation than they have received. *Testimonies for the Church*, vol. 7, 63.

The Lord would have His people come to Him for their power of healing. He will baptize them with His Holy Spirit, and fit them for a service that will make them a blessing in restoring the spiritual and physical health of those who need healing. Ibid., vol. 9, 178.

But few can take a course of training in our medical institutions. But all can study our health literature, and become intelligent on this important subject. *Medical Ministry*, 320.

Many will go out to labor for the Master who have not been able to take a regular course of study in school. God will help these workers. They will obtain knowledge from the higher school. *Special Testimonies*, Series B, 214–215.

THOSE who have formal training in the spiritual and the health fields can certainly aid lay workers in becoming effective medical missionaries.

There are those who with a few months' instruction would be prepared to go out and do acceptable medical missionary work. *The Paulson Collection of Ellen G. White Letters*, 38.

Christian Philanthropists

SOME MAY wonder how God can expect, much less require, all his workers and church members to combine both spiritual and health work in their efforts for others. It certainly will not be possible without special effort, but neither is it as impossible as it first seems. To begin with, all who have the hope of eternal life must first be knowledgeable of and then must practice in their own lives the spiritual and the physical laws which govern their being. They will not only be enthusiastic health reformers and commandment-keeping Christians, they will also have firsthand experience in the use of nature's remedies for the treatment of disease. This basic spiritual and health information and personal practice required of all Christ's followers will fit and inspire them to share this knowledge with others. Thus lay workers will be easily equipped to function effectively in health education, home healthcare, and in encouraging and motivating their fellow beings to make necessary changes in physical and spiritual habits. Those with professional training in health work will be able to add modern therapeutics, if indicated, to this same basic work. God requires each of us to share that which we must already have for our own personal physical and spiritual health. In this way God's health system provides a large body of trained, highly motivated health workers equipped to work in the areas of health preservation, home care, mental hygiene, and health behavior change—the very areas in which other health systems fail the most.

> Intelligent, self-denying, self-sacrificing men are now needed,—men who realize the solemnity and importance of God's work, and who as Christian philanthropists will fulfill the commission of Christ. The medical missionary work given us to do, means something to every one of us. It is a work of soul saving; it is the proclamation of the gospel message. *Review and Herald*, vol. 6, 441.

Heaven's Financial Methods

GOD'S MEDICAL missionary workers are not only different from those of the world, and doing a work different from those of the world, but they are working on a different financial basis from those of the world. This factor is important in making God's method more economical than that of other systems. It is also essential in representing Christ's earthly work. God's professional health workers are to be bound to His organizational work the same as all other workers and all are to be paid on the same scale. Those who work to heal the body should not make a profit from sins effects any more than do those who work to heal the soul.

> The gospel of Christ is to be bound up with medical missionary work, and medical missionary work is to be bound up with the gospel ministry. The world needs the efforts of medical missionaries who are bound up with the gospel message. *Medical Ministry*, 252.

> Medical missionary work is not to be drawn apart and made

separate from church organization. *Testimonies for the Church*, vol. 8, 164.

COUNSEL to a physician in perplexity follows:

You are not to set up in business for yourself. This is not the Lord's plan. You are not to unite with unbelievers in medical work. Neither is this the Lord's plan. *Medical Ministry*, 45.

My brother, the Lord needs your help in His work. Will you not be His helping hand? It would be a serious mistake for you to accept a worldly position, where it would not be possible for you to do the medical missionary work that God desires you to do. Do not make this mistake. Ibid., 47–48.

THERE is also counsel for teachers of medical missionaries:

Temptations will come to you to think that in order to carry forward the medical missionary work you must stand aloof from church organization or church discipline. To stand thus would place you on an unsound footing. The work done for those who come to you for instruction is not complete unless they are educated to work in connection with the church. *Counsels on Health*, 523.

COUNSEL in regard to salary follows:

Let not the idea prevail for a moment that man's power to command high wages is a measure of his value in the sight of God as a worker. *Selected Messages*, book 2, 193.

Some would follow a worldly fashion in the drawing of their salaries; but the Lord does not view matters as these men view them. He views our duties and responsibilities in the light of Christ's self-denying example. Ibid., 198.

The charges made by other practicing physicians are not to be his criterion. The diseased bodies over which he works are God's property. *Medical Ministry*, 121.

We are not to let the wage question stand in the way of our responding to the call of duty, wherever our service may be required. The Lord can bring matters around so that a blessing will attach to our labors far exceeding any compensation we may or may not receive. *Selected Messages*, book 2, 205.

Why should the Christian physician, who is believing, expecting, looking, waiting, and longing for the coming kingdom of Christ, when sickness and death will no longer have power over the saints, expect more pay for his services than the Christian editor or the Christian minister? He may say that his work is more wearing. That is yet to be proved. Let him work as he can endure it, and not violate the laws of life which he teaches to his patients. There are no good reasons why he should overwork and receive large pay for it, more than the minister or editor. *Testimonies for the Church*, vol. 1, 640.

Our physicians need to reform in the matter of making high charges for critical operations. And the reform should extend farther than this. Often an exorbitant fee is charged for even small services, because physicians are supposed to be governed in their charges by the practices of worldly physicians. There are those who follow worldly policy in order to accumulate means, as they say, for God's service. But God does not accept such offerings. He says, "I hate robbery for burnt offering." Isaiah 61:8, *The Kress Collection*, 59.

PROFESSIONAL medical missionaries, having bound themselves in medical missionary work to the organization and its pay scale, are to receive their salary from the tithe just as the ministers.

Some, who do not see the advantage of educating the youth to be physicians both of the mind and of the body, say that the tithe should not be used to support medical missionaries who devote their time to treating the sick. In response to such statements as these, I am instructed to say that the mind must not become so narrowed down that it cannot take in the truth of the situation. A minister of the gospel, who is also a medical missionary, who can cure physical ailments, is a much more efficient worker than one who can not do this. His work as a minister of the gospel is much more complete. *Medical Ministry*, 245.

Volunteer Work

ASIDE from the health work done by those who live from this work, there will be a large amount of work done in the health field without fees or salaries. There will be a large group of volunteers sharing what they know and what they have experienced out of love for their fellow beings and their Creator.

As they see one with no inducement of earthly praise or compensation come into their wretched homes, ministering to the sick, feeding the hungry, clothing the naked, and tenderly pointing all to Him of whose love and pity the human worker is but the messenger,—as they see this, their hearts are touched. Gratitude springs up. Faith is kindled. They see that God cares for them; and they are prepared to listen as His word is opened. *Testimonies for the Church*, vol. 6, 259.

Heaven's Health Institutions

IN GOD'S war against disease, He has designated certain types of facilities as being best suited for His purposes. These facilities, as does the rest of God's plan, are to differ from those normally used in other health programs. It is of great importance to the success of God's plan that we understand well the purposes of His institutions. Other approaches to the problem of disease may utilize types of institutions different from those God has proposed for His health program, but His purposes and His plans for His work do not change.

The purpose of our health institutions is not first and foremost to be that of hospitals. *Medical Ministry*, 27–28.

We never proposed to establish sanitariums to have them run in nearly the same grooves as other institutions. If we do not have a sanitarium which is, in many things, decidedly contrary to other institutions, we can see nothing gained. *Spalding and Magan Collection*, 45.

From the light I have received, I know that if ever there was a country where a sanitarium was needed it is New South

Wales, and I may say also, Victoria. There is indeed a great necessity for such an institution. The people say, "But we have our hospitals." Some may go to the hospitals and get benefit from the treatments, but it would mean death for others to go there. We should have a sanitarium under our own regulations, that the truth of God on health reform may be given to the world. Those connected with such an institution, who are being educated as nurses, should be trained to go forth from the institution as solid as a rock upon the principles of health reform and other points of the truth. *(Australasian) Union Conference Record*, 12.

HEAVEN'S health institutions should be centers where the sick are treated and by their treatment enabled better to utilize spiritual truths. Caregivers in these institutions will both practice and promulgate the knowledge of nature's laws of disease prevention and of nature's simple remedies. The purpose for these institutions will be to aid people to so completely in harmony with nature, and nature's God, that He will be able to restore them eternally to the society of His unfallen creation.

God would have a health institution established which will in its influence be closely connected with the closing work for mortals fitting for immortality. . . . The great object of this institution would be to improve the health of the body that the afflicted may more highly appreciate eternal things. *Testimonies for the Church*, vol. 1, 564.

A work of reformation is to be carried on in our institutions. Physicians, workers, nurses are to realize that they are on probation, on trial for their present life, and for that life which measures with the life of God. We are to put every faculty to the stretch in order to bring saving truths to the attention of suffering human beings. This must be done in connection with the work of healing the sick. Ibid., vol. 6, 253.

I have been instructed that our medical institutions are to stand as witnesses for God. They are established to relieve the sick and the afflicted, to awaken a spirit of inquiry, to disseminate light, and to advance reform. These institutions, rightly conducted, will be the means of bringing a knowledge of the reforms essential to prepare a people for the coming of the Lord, before many that otherwise, it would be impossible for us to reach. Ibid., vol. 7, 104.

This institution is designed of God to be one of the greatest aids in preparing a people to be perfect before God. Ibid., vol. 3, 166.

In all our health institutions, it should be made a special feature of the work to give instruction in regard to the laws of health. The principles of health reform should be carefully and thoroughly set before all, both patients and helpers. This work requires moral courage; for while many will profit by such efforts, others will be offended. *Counsels on Health*, 452.

I was shown that we should provide a home for the afflicted and those who wish to learn how to take care of their bodies that they may prevent sickness. *Testimonies for the Church*, vol. 1, 485–486.

If we are to go to the expense of building sanitariums in order that we may work for the salvation of the sick and afflicted, we must plan our work in such a way that those we desire to help will receive the help they need. We are to do all in our power for the healing of the body; but we are to make the healing of the soul of far greater importance. Those who come to our sanitariums as patients are to be shown the way of salvation, that they may repent and hear the words: Thy sins are forgiven thee; go in peace, and sin no more. Ibid., vol. 7, 96.

Institutional Workers

WITH UNDERSTANDING of God's clearly expressed purposes for His healthcare institutions comes insight regarding the type of workers that He requires for these institutions. An institution's success depends largely upon its workers, and it cannot provide that which its workers do not personally possess and share. The purposes and practices of any institution are determined by the sum of the purposes and practices of its individual workers.

Let our sanitariums become what they should be, homes where healing is ministered to sin-sick souls. And this will be done when the workers have a living connection with the Great Healer. *Counsels on Health*, 542.

Those who have no burning desire to save souls are not the ones who should connect with our sanitariums. *Medical Ministry*, 191.

I was shown that physicians and helpers should be of the highest order, those who have an experimental knowledge of the truth, who will command respect and whose word can be relied on. *Testimonies for the Church*, vol. 1, 567.

Every physician in our ranks should be a Christian. Only those physicians who are genuine Bible Christians can discharge aright the high duties of their profession. Ibid., vol. 6, 229.

Better for the work to go crippled than for workers who are not fully devoted to be employed. *Medical Ministry*, 207.

Neither physicians nor helpers should attempt to perform their work without taking time to pray. *Testimonies for the Church*, vol. 4, 560.

A special effort should be made to secure the services of conscientious, Christian workers. It is the purpose of God that a health institution should be organized and controlled exclusively by Seventh-day Adventists; and when unbelievers are brought in to occupy responsible positions, an influence is presiding there that will tell with great weight against the sanitarium. God did not intend that this institution should be carried on after the order of any other health institute in the land; but that it should be one of the most effectual instrumentalities in his hands of giving light to the world. It should stand forth with scientific ability, with moral and spiritual power, and as a faithful sentinel of reform in all its bearings; and all who act a part in it should be reformers, having respect to its rules, and heeding the light of health reform now shining upon us as a people. Ibid., vol. 4, 556.

Institutional Location

THE PURPOSE for a health institution will influence where it is located. In order for the sick to recover, they should be removed as far as possible from environmental factors detrimental to physical, mental and spiritual health. They should be placed as close as possible to the environmental agents conducive to health. Thus God's health institutions are to be located in a natural setting close to nature's God, from whence cometh healing power.

Let us learn from Him not to choose for our sanitariums the places most agreeable to our taste, but those places best suited to our work. Light has been given me that in medical missionary work we have lost great advantages by failing to realize the need of a change in our plans in regard to the location of sanitariums. It is the Lord's will that these institutions shall be situated in the country, in the midst of surroundings as attractive as possible. In nature, the Lord's garden, the sick will always find something to divert their attention from themselves and lift their thoughts to God. *Testimonies for the Church*, vol. 7, 80.

Thus, though we are removed from the cities twenty or thirty miles, we shall be able to reach the people, and those who desire health will have opportunity to regain it under conditions most favorable. *Counsels on Health*, 172.

The more closely His plan of life is followed, the more wonderfully will He work to restore suffering humanity. The sick need to be brought into close touch with nature. *The Ministry of Healing*, 261.

WE ARE to locate small health institutions with our schools, with mutual benefit as the results.

Small local sanitariums are to be established in connection with our schools. *Medical Ministry*, 156.

There is a sanitarium a few miles from here. The two institutions can work together harmoniously. *Pacific Union Recorder*, October 7, 1909, 272.

I am thankful when I think of the advantages enjoyed by the schools that are established near our sanitariums, so that the work of the two educational institutions can blend. The students in these schools, while gaining an education in the knowledge of present truth, can also learn how to be ministers of healing to those whom they go forth to serve. *Counsels on Health*, 542.

City Centers

THE COUNTRY-located schools and sanitariums are to serve as outposts for work in the cities.

The cities are to be worked from outposts. Said the messenger of God, "Shall not the cities be warned? Yes, not by God's people living in them, but by their visiting them, to warn them of what is coming upon the earth. *Evangelism*, 77.

It is God's design that our people should locate outside the cities, and from these outposts warn the cities, and raise in them memorials for God. There must be a force of influence in the cities, that the message of warning shall be heard. Ibid., 76.

CITY CENTERS, operated from the country outpost centers, are to include a variety of endeavors. These will serve as feeders for the country sanitariums.

I have been given light that in many cities it is advisable for a restaurant to be connected with treatment rooms. The two can cooperate in upholding right principles. In connection with these it is sometimes advisable to have rooms that will serve as lodgings for the sick. These establishments will serve as feeders to the sanitariums located in the country and would better be conducted in rented buildings. We are not to erect in the cities large buildings in which to care for the sick, because God has plainly indicated that the sick can be better cared for outside of the cities. In many places it will be necessary to begin sanitarium work in the cities; but, as much as possible, this work should be transferred to the country as soon as suitable locations can be secured. *Testimonies for the Church*, vol. 7, 55.

FACILITIES for conducting cooking schools are to be associated with restaurants and treatment rooms.

> Wherever medical missionary work is carried on in our large cities, cooking schools should be held; and wherever a strong educational missionary work is in progress, a hygienic restaurant of some sort should be established, which shall give a practical illustration of the proper selection and the healthful preparation of foods. Ibid., 55.

> Hygienic restaurants are to be established in the cities, and by them the message of temperance is to be proclaimed. Arrangements should be made to hold meetings in connection with our restaurants. Whenever possible, let a room be provided where the patrons can be invited to lectures on the science of health and Christian temperance, where they can receive instruction on the preparation of wholesome food and on other important subjects. *Counsels on Health*, 481.

HEALTH food stores are to be associated with these centers of influence in the cities.

> Centers of influence may be established in many places by the opening up of health food stores, hygienic restaurants, and treatment rooms. Not all that needs to be done can be specified before a beginning is made. *Testimonies for the Church*, vol. 7, 234.

Size and Number of Institutions

THE LORD'S Health Work is not to be limited to a few localities. It is to be conducted throughout the whole world. God requests that small institutions be established in many places. Keeping them small will help them maintain a proper atmosphere.

> The proclamation of the truth in all parts of the world calls for small sanitariums in many places, not in the heart of cities, but in places where city influences will be as little felt as possible. *Medical Ministry*, 159.

Sanitariums are to be established all through our world, and managed by a people who are in harmony with God's laws, a people who will cooperate with God in advocating the truth that determines the case of every soul for whom Christ died. Ibid., 25–26.

For many years light has been given that sanitariums should be established near every large city. Ibid., 326

It is not the Lord's will for His people to erect mammoth sanitariums anywhere. Many sanitariums are to be established. They are not to be large, but sufficiently complete to do a good and successful work. . . . Never are we to rely upon worldly recognition and rank. Never are we, in the establishment of institutions to try to compete with worldly institutions in size or splendor. *Testimonies for the Church*, vol. 7, 100.

It is almost impossible to find talent to manage a large sanitarium as it should be managed. The workers are not all under the control of the Spirit of God, as they should be, and a worldly spirit comes in. Ibid., 60.

The Benefits of Right Doing

WE HAVE mentioned the fact that once the ill are relieved from suffering they are more susceptible to spiritual truths and are more capable of comprehending and obeying them. Thus, one of God's prime purposes for establishing a health program is the promulgation and the acceptance of spiritual truth. Physical health is conducive to spiritual health. The reverse being also true, spiritual health is highly conducive to physical health; therefore instruction in religious truths is very important to the success of Heaven's Health Program. Much tact should be used in presenting controversial points, but the knowledge of a sin-pardoning, loving Saviour is always of benefit to the sick.

The consciousness of right doing is the best medicine for diseased bodies and minds. *Counsels on Health*, 628.

Many are suffering from maladies of the soul far more than from diseases of the body, and they will find no relief until they come to Christ, the wellspring of life. The burden of sin, with its unrest and unsatisfied desires, lies at the foundation of a large share of the maladies the sinner suffers. Ibid., 502.

The love which Christ diffuses through the whole being is a vitalizing power. Every vital part—the brain, the heart, the nerves—it touches with healing. By it the highest energies of the being are aroused to activity. It frees the soul from the guilt and sorrow, the anxiety and care, that crush the life forces. With it come serenity and composure. It implants in the soul joy that nothing earthly can destroy—joy in the Holy Spirit—health giving, life-giving joy. *The Ministry of Healing*, 115.

Satan's Interference

A S PREVIOUSLY mentioned, whoever sincerely attempts to develop or operate an effective health program has the devil to fight. Unfortunately the devil is more real than many in the health field realize. He is the primary cause of disease and suffering. He is the destroyer. He has palmed off on mankind the idea that man evolved from lower life-forms and has a body possessing great adaptability. Believing that there is no Creator, man assumes that neither are there fixed rules of life, either spiritual or physical. As long as he believes thus, Satan does not care how much "spirituality" or "health" a man enjoys. Satan's real concern is that man does not form a connection with Heaven's Spiritual or Health Programs. He is not too worried when scientists discover some of the laws of health, so long as these laws are not recognized as originating with a loving Creator. Especially does Satan not want man to know that this loving Creator has revealed the principles or laws governing man's physical and spiritual health, both for this life and for eternity. He does not want mankind to know that we were created in the image of God, to be temples of His Holy Spirit, and that we are to glorify our Maker. He does not want health reform to be promulgated or for man to realize that he is required by his Creator to give an account for the care he gives his body temple.

SATAN has filled the world with superstitions and irrational approaches to disease and even where rational methods are used, he does all in his power to prevent them from being allied with the message of health reform and nature's remedies. In the Garden of Eden, Satan first planted the idea that longevity is not affected by what you eat, and he still quite successfully maintains that obedience to God's revealed will is not essential to success in the field of health. The majority want to live as they please and they expect the health worker to prevent or counteract the results. Modern therapeutics can be interpreted to lend credence to Satan's claims. Modern science has found rational approaches to disease so effective that many feel that health reform and nature's simple remedies are not as essential as they used to be. Whoever approaches the problem of disease, neglecting health reform or nature's remedies will find in the long-run that they were providing only a palliative and thus a deceptive form of healthcare.

> The very last deception of Satan will be to make of none effect the testimony of the Spirit of God. "Where there is no vision, the people perish" (Proverbs 29:18). Satan will work ingeniously, in different ways and through different agencies, to unsettle the confidence of God's remnant people in the true testimony. *Selected Messages*, book 2, 78.

> The human family is suffering because of the transgression of the laws of God. Satan is constantly urging men to accept his principles, and thus he is seeking to counterwork the work of God. . . .The Lord desires through His people, to answer Satan's charges by showing the result of obedience to right principles. *Medical Ministry*, 187.

AS A PEOPLE, we must guard against participating in a health program which does not place strong emphasis upon obedience to God's expressed will as a requisite to true and lasting health.

> The Lord has shown me that if the enemy can by any means divert the work into wrong channels, and thus hinder its advancement, he will do so. *Testimonies for the Church*, vol. 8, 182.

It is the plan and constant effort of Satan to entangle the work of God in a supposed beneficent and excellent work so that doors cannot be opened to enter new fields. *Temperance*, 222.

FAILURE TO follow God's directions will lead to serious consequences.

Conformity to the world is causing many of our people to lose their bearings. I feel deeply over this matter, because it is continually kept before me by the Lord. For many years it has been presented to me again and again that a worldly policy has been coming into the management of many of our institutions. And when I read the published Testimonies that were given in the early seventies and even before that time, I am surprised to see how clearly our dangers in this matter have been pointed out, and how plainly the right way has been outlined from the beginning. But the way, so plainly specified, has not been followed. Men act as if counsels had never been given; and yet we expect the Lord to uplift us and to do great things for us! True, He will help us if we so relate ourselves to Him that He can; but He will not serve with us while we are weaving threads of selfishness into the web. *Manuscript Releases*, volume 1, 243.

The medical missionary work should be a part of the work of every church in our land. Disconnected from the church it would soon become a strange medley of disorganized atoms. It would consume, but not produce. Instead of acting as God's helping hand to forward His truth, it would sap the life and force from the church and weaken the message. Conducted independently, it would not only consume talent and means needed in other lines, but in the very work of helping the helpless apart from the ministry of the word, it would place men where they would scoff at Bible truth. *Testimonies for the Church*, vol. 6, 289.

The Effectiveness of Heaven's Plan

M ANY ARE aware that Heaven's Health Service will be one
hundred percent effective in the earth made new, but they question how effective it can be in this present life. It is true that God will
never remove all disease and pain until sin is permanently eradicated. God's health program, however, can be very successful even
in this present life. A report has been made of a study in California
involving fifty thousand people. Results showed that Seventh-day
Adventist men between the ages of thirty-five and forty years had a
six and two-tenths-year life expectancy advantage over non-Adventist
males of the same age. This remarkable benefit was accomplished in
spite of the fact that only about fifty percent of the Adventists were
attempting to live up to the health reform message. (Nelson and
VanDolson, op. cit., 17–18).

> Ye said also, Behold what a weariness is it! and ye have snuffed
> at it, saith the Lord of Hosts: and ye brought that which was torn,
> and the lame, and the sick; thus ye brought an offering: should I
> accept this of your hand? saith the Lord. Malachi 1:13.

> If the sick and suffering will do only as well as they know in
> regard to living out the principles of health reform perseveringly,
> then they will in nine cases out of ten recover from their ail-
> ments. *Medical Ministry*, 224.

T HIS STATEMENT is very remarkable and exciting. Thus true
health reform—conformity to nature's laws—is a very highly effective therapeutic agent. It should also be just as effective in preventing disease as it is in aiding recovery. We are told that ninety percent
of those whose lives are in peril from disease will be benefited by
the knowledge of a sin-pardoning Saviour.

> He [the God-fearing physician] should not listen to the sug-
> gestion that it is dangerous to speak of their eternal interests to
> those whose lives are in peril, lest it should make them worse;
> for in nine cases out of ten the knowledge of a sin-pardoning
> Saviour would make them better both in mind and body. Jesus
> can limit the power of Satan. He is the physician in whom the
> sin-sick soul may trust to heal the maladies of the body as well

as of the soul. *Testimonies for the Church*, vol. 5, 449.

IMPROVEMENT of health while on this earth can be very remarkable according to the following statements.

> But if all would seek to become intelligent in regard to their bodily necessities, sickness would be rare instead of common. An ounce of prevention is worth a pound of cure. *Selected Messages*, book 2, 291.

> If the living machinery were properly cared for, there would not be today one-thousandth part of the suffering that there is. We are God's children, and we are to be apt students in studying the philosophy of health. If we are well, we should learn how to keep well by studying to some purpose the principles of health reform. Seventh-day Adventists should not follow the health-destroying customs of the world because it is the fashion to follow these customs. *Manuscript Releases*, volume two, 181.

> By His own working agencies He has created material which will restore the sick to health. If men would use aright the wisdom God has given them, this world would be a place resembling heaven. *Medical Ministry*, 121.

THE ABOVE statements give us thoughts to ponder. How weighty are the responsibilities of God's people!

The Impact on the Workers

OBEDIENCE to Heaven's plan will also have a great effect upon God's people, aside from improved physical health. They will become much more effective workers for God.

> If Seventh-day Adventists practiced what they profess to believe, if they were sincere health reformers, they would indeed be a spectacle to the world, to angels, and to men. And they would show a far greater zeal for the salvation of those who are ignorant of the truth. *Counsels on Health*, 575.

If the church would manifest a greater interest in the reforms [on health] which God Himself has brought to them to fit
them for His coming, their influence would be tenfold what it
now is. *Testimonies for the Church*, vol, 3, 171.

Relations Between Prevention and Acute Care

THERE is much discussion as to how emphasis should be distributed among the various approaches to disease. The conventional
approach to disease—detection of its cause and its removal if possible—has many advocates. Many feel, however, that the main hope
for success lies in the endeavor to prevent the disease in the first
place. Joseph Malines has authored a poem which expresses very
clearly the feelings of this latter group.

"The Fence or the Ambulance?"

Twas a dangerous cliff, as they freely confessed.
   Though to walk near its crest was so pleasant:
But over its terrible edge there had slipped
   A duke and many a peasant;
So the people said something would have to be done,
   But their projects did not at all tally:
Some said, "Put a fence around the edge of the cliff";
   Some, "An ambulance down in the valley."

But the cry for the ambulance carried the day,
   For it spread to the neighboring city;
A fence may be useful or not, it is true,
   But each heart became brimful of pity
For those who had slipped o'er that dangerous cliff,
   And the dwellers in highway and alley
Gave pounds or gave pence, not to put up a fence,
   But an ambulance in the valley.

"For the cliff is all right if you're careful," they said,

"And if folks even slip or are dropping,
It isn't the slipping that hurts them so much
   As the shock down below-when they're stopping,"
So day after day when these mishaps occurred,
   Quick forth would the rescuers sally
To pick up the victims who fell off the cliff
   With their ambulance down in the valley.

Then an old man remarked: "It's a marvel to me
   That people give far more attention
To repairing results than to stopping the cause,
   When they's much better aim at prevention.
Let us stop at its source all this mischief," cried he,
   Come, neighbors and friends, let us rally;
If the cliff we will fence, we might almost dispense
   With the ambulance down in the valley."

Oh, he's a fanatic," the others rejoined;
   "Dispense with the ambulance? Never!
He'd dispense with all charities, too, if he could:
   No, no! We'll support them forever.
Aren't we picking up folks just as fast as they fall?
   And shall this man dictate to us? Shall he?
Why should people of sense stop to put a fence
   While their ambulance works in the valley?"

Thus this story so old has beautifully told
   How our people, with best of intentions,
Have wasted their years and lavished their tears
   On treatment, with naught for prevention.

But a sensible few, who are practical, too,
   Will not bear with such nonsense much longer;
They believe that prevention is better than cure,
   And their party will soon be the stronger.
Encourage them, then, with your purse, voice, and pen,
   And (while other philanthropists dally)
They will scorn all pretence, and put up a stout fence
   On the cliff that hangs over the valley.

DOES GOD'S health plan place emphasis primarily upon prevention or upon acute care? Before sin entered the garden of Eden, Adam and Eve maintained their God-given health by obedience to the laws of health and by partaking of the tree of life. Their obedience prevented disease. The emphasis before sin entered was upon health preservation—disease prevention. In God's dealings with the children of Israel, the emphasis was upon disease prevention by health education and sanitation. When Christ was upon earth, He provided much acute care but it was associated with the admonition to "go and sin no more," which was preventive care. We are told that whole villages were without anyone sick after His passing through. From this statement, one might get the idea that God's emphasis is primarily upon acute care. However, we must remember that Christ's healing of the people was associated with the preaching of "the kingdom of heaven is at hand" and was thus symbolic of when His kingdom will really come and again, by His miraculous power, all will be healed. When perfect health is again restored to mankind, it will again be preserved and disease prevented by obedience to nature's laws and by access to the tree of life. Thus the ideal approach to disease is preventive. This side of heaven there will always be a place and need to raise the fallen, but the emphasis must be on the "go and sin no more."

> The object of the health reform and the Health Institute is not, like a dose of "Pain Killer" or "Instant Relief," to quiet the pains of to-day. No indeed! Its great object is to teach the people how to live so as to give nature a chance to remove and resist disease. *Testimonies for the Church*, vol. 1, 643.

> The distinction between prevention and cure has not been made sufficiently important. Teach the people that it is better to know how to keep well than how to cure disease. *Medical Ministry*, 221.

> The first labors of a physician should be to educate the sick and suffering in the very course they should pursue to prevent disease. The greatest good can be done by our trying to enlighten the minds of all we can obtain access to as to the best course for them to pursue to prevent sickness and suffering, and broken constitutions, and premature death. *Selected Messages*, book 2, 282.

THUS IF the knowledge of health reform, with its potential ninety-percent effectiveness, in association with knowledge of nature's true remedies, was widely known and faithfully utilized, one can imagine how much less demand there would be for acute care. A properly informed, properly motivated, and properly empowered lay public would go a long way in solving the health problems of our day.

———————

Part III

The Role and Response of Christ's Followers

A Special Task

WE AS A people have been chosen by God to carry to the world the last warning message. The message is referred to as the three angels' messages. It emphasizes that God's judgment has arrived and that man is to give glory to his Creator by obedience to His laws of health and to His moral law.

> For His church in every generation God has a special truth and a special work. *Christ's Object Lessons*, 78.

IT HAS previously been pointed out how health reform is an integral and essential part of the third angel's message.

> In a special sense Seventh-day Adventists have been set in the world as watchmen and light-bearers. To them has been entrusted the last warning for a perishing world. On them is shining wonderful light from the Word of God. They have been given a work of the most solemn import, the proclamation of the first, second, and third angel's messages. There is no other work of so great importance. They are to allow nothing else to absorb their attention. *Testimonies for the Church*, vol. 9, 19.

IN THE organization of any program it is essential that specially prepared people be charged with specified, special duties. For any plan to have success the proper people must be in their proper places doing the proper work. Thus God has organized His plan against disease. In these last decades He has given men of the world marvelous insight and knowledge in order to develop the modern therapeutics. This ability and duty has been assigned primarily to the world. This task they can do. However, there is a work against disease which the world cannot do and this ability and duty God has given to His chosen people. It involves practicing and teaching obedience to His laws as found in the human body as a moral obligation to present the temple of God to Him as a living sacrifice to glorify Him. This message is to be given to every nation, tongue, and people. It involves emphasis upon true preventive medicine, joined to a spiritual awakening. Such a task the world cannot do.

That thy way may be known upon earth, thy saving health among all nations. Psalm 67:2.

God has committed to us a special work, a work that no other people can do. He has promised us the aid of His Holy Spirit. The heavenly current is flowing earthward for the accomplishment of the very work appointed us. Let not this heavenly current be turned aside by our deviations from the straightforward path marked out by Christ. *Testimonies for the Church*, vol. 6, 244.

As a people we have been given the work of making known the principles of health reform. *Counsels on Health*, 443.

We have been given the work of advancing health reform. The Lord desires His people to be in harmony with one another. As you must know, we shall not leave the position in which, for the last thirty-five years, the Lord has been bidding us stand. *Medical Ministry*, 279.

The work of promulgating the principles of health reform which the Lord has outlined to us must be accomplished. *Medical Ministry*, 60.

If the Lord's workers take up lines of labor which crowd out that which should be done by them in communicating light to the world, God does not receive through their labors the glory that should accrue to His holy name. When God calls a man to do a certain work in His cause, He does not also lay upon him burdens that other men can and should bear. *Testimonies for the Church*, vol. 6, 245.

The Lord has marked out our way of working. As a people we are not to imitate and fall in with Salvation Army methods. This is not the work that the Lord has given us to do. Neither is it our work to condemn them and speak harsh words against them. There are precious, self-sacrificing souls in the Salvation Army. We are to treat them kindly. There are in the Army honest souls, who are sincerely serving the Lord and who will see greater light, advancing to the acceptance of all truth. The Salvation Army workers are trying to save the neglected, downtrodden ones. Discourage them not. Let them do that class of work by their own methods and in their own way. But the Lord has plainly pointed out the work that Seventh-day Adventists are to do. Ibid., vol. 8, 184–185.

To care for these needy ones is a good work; yet in this age of the world the Lord does not give us as a people directions to establish large and expensive institutions for this purpose. If, however, there are among us individuals who feel called of God to establish institutions for the care of orphan children, let them follow out their convictions of duty. But in caring for the world's poor they should appeal to the world for support. They are not to draw upon the people to whom the Lord has given the most important work ever given to men, the work of bringing the last message of mercy before all nations, kindreds, tongues, and people. The Lord's treasury must have a surplus to sustain the work of the gospel in "regions beyond." Ibid., vol. 6, 286.

When freedom was proclaimed to the captives, [slaves in the southern United States] a favorable time was given in which to establish schools, and to teach the people to take care of themselves. Much of this kind of work was done by various denominations, and God honored their work. *Review and Herald*, vol. 3, 317–318.

THUS GOD has assigned to His people definite areas of labor in His Health program. Obedience to God's spiritual and physical laws is the great testing truth for mankind. His final movement has been given the special task of promulgating that portion of His health program which determines man's eternal destiny. The world can and should do the palliative work but our emphasis must be upon the truly curative. The world can provide temporal health, but only His people can offer eternal health. Eternity will judge as to which is the more important and the more compassionate. God cannot give an immortal body to one who has not shown a desire to do all in his power to preserve the health of his present body.

> He that is faithful in that which is least is faithful also in much; and he that is unjust in the least is unjust also in much. Luke 16:10.

Concentrated Effort

OURS IS a great and immense task. It is worldwide in scope. As a comparatively small people, success in our task will require activation and concentration of all our manpower and material resources. There is no excess for doing that which is not essential to our task.

> Christ says: "Where Satan has set his throne, there shall stand My cross. Satan shall be cast out, and I will be lifted up to draw all men unto Me. I will become the center of the redeemed world. ... I will engage every sanctified human agency in the universe. None of My agencies are to be absent. I have work for all who love Me, employment for every soul who will work under My direction. The activity of Satan's army, the danger that surrounds the human soul calls for the energies of every worker. *Testimonies for the Church*, vol. 6, 237.

> Heavenly angels have long been waiting for human agents-the members of the church-to cooperate with them in the great work to be done. They are waiting for you. So vast is the field, so comprehensive the design, that every sanctified heart will be pressed into service as an instrument of divine power. Ibid., vol. 9, 46.

> Man is measured by his consecration and faithfulness in working out the will of God. If the remnant people of God will walk before Him in humility of faith, He will carry out through them His eternal purpose, enabling them to work harmoniously in giving to the world the truth as it is in Jesus. He will use all, men, women, and children, in making the light shine forth to the world, and calling out a people that will be true to His commandments. *The Paulson Collection of Ellen G. White Letters*, 284.

GOD HAS placed every believer under tribute to work for Him.

The whole treasure of heaven is at our command in our work of preparing the way of the Lord. God has made it possible by giving us the cooperation of heavenly angels, for our work to be a wonderful, yes, a glorious success. But success will seldom result from scattered, individual effort. The influence of every church member is required. The influence of ministers and workers is needed to prepare the way for the light and glory of God. Every soul who claims to believe in Jesus, God lays under tribute to Himself. *Ellen G. White, 1888 Materials*, 746.

The Spirit of Reformers

OURS IS a task primarily of reform and thus it behooves us to know in what spirit we can best aid others to reform. How can we help them to change their physical and spiritual ways of life?

Of all people in the world, reformers should be the most unselfish, the most kind, the most courteous. In their lives should be seen the true goodness of unselfish deeds. The worker who manifests a lack of courtesy, who shows impatience at the ignorance or waywardness of others, who speaks hastily or acts thoughtlessly, may close the door to hearts so that he can never reach them. *The Ministry of Healing*, 157.

Not words, but deeds. The daily life tells much more than any number of words. A uniform cheerfulness, tender kindness, Christian benevolence, patience, and love will melt away prejudice, and open the heart to the reception of the truth. Few understand the power of these precious influences. *Evangelism*, 543.

Reformers are not destroyers. They will never seek to ruin those who do not harmonize with their plans and assimilate to them. Reformers must advance, not retreat. They must be decided, firm, resolute, unflinching; but firmness must not degenerate into a domineering spirit. God desires to have all who serve Him firm as a rock where principle is concerned, but meek and lowly of heart, as was Christ. Then, abiding in Christ, they can do the work He would do, were He in their place.

Testimonies for the Church, vol. 6, 151.

The Lord's Methods

TO DO THE Lord's work is to do His work in His way. The modern tendency is to "Do my thing in my way" but God requires workers for Him to do things His way. Any other way, sooner or later, will meet with failure.

Unless the Lord builds the house, those who build it labor in vain. Psalm 127:1, RSV.

GOD HAS revealed to His people the general outline of His work and He asks that His workers use all of their knowledge and wisdom in carrying out their tasks. He has promised daily guidance to guarantee our success. But to begin with, we must be sure we start with God's plan. Then man can bring to the work only his wisdom and knowledge which is in harmony with and additive to God's previously revealed will. Any future guidance from God will also be in harmony with His previously revealed will. Thus we must build on a firm foundation. We must be specialists in the counsel of God which pertains to our area of work as found in the Bible and the Spirit of Prophecy. Only thus can we be sure we are actually involved in doing God's work.

There are many ways of practicing the healing art; but there is only one way that Heaven approves. *Testimonies for the Church*, vol. 5, 443.

Heaven is worth everything to us. We must not run any risk in this matter. We must know that our steps are ordered by the Lord. *Temperance*, 114.

We are God's servants, and we are to be workers together with Him, doing His work in His way, that all for whom we labor may see that our desire is to reach a higher standard of holiness. *Testimonies for the Church*, vol. 7, 96.

For years the Lord has had a controversy with His people

because they have followed their own judgment, and have not relied on divine wisdom. Let the workers take heed lest they get in the Lord's way, hindering the advancement of His work, thinking that their wisdom is sufficient for the successful planning and carrying forward of the work. If they do this, the Lord will correct their error. By His divine Spirit He enlightens and trains His workers. He shapes His own providences to carry forward His work according to His mind and will. Ibid., vol. 8, 186.

The Lord God of Israel would not have given directions to have everything according to the pattern shown in the mount if He had not meant us to work according to those directions. *(Australasian) Union Conference Record*, 12.

God's Instructions Unchanged

My covenant will I not break, nor alter the thing that is gone out of my lips. Psalm 89:34.

So shall my word be that goeth forth out of my mouth; it shall not return unto me void, but it shall accomplish that which I please, and it shall prosper in the thing whereto I sent it. Isaiah 55:11.

IF WE WORK according to God's plan, we can expect God's daily guidance and protection and He will add to us still greater truths. Our message of health will be a growing message, but its previously revealed principles will not be negated by God.

I know that whatsoever God doeth, it shall be for ever: nothing can be put to it nor anything taken from it and God doeth it that men should fear before Him. Ecclesiastes 3:14.

We cannot afford to neglect one ray of light God has given. *Spalding and Magan Collection*, 7.

And thine ears shall hear a word behind thee, saying, This is the way, walk ye in it, when ye turn to the right hand, and when ye turn to the left. Isaiah 30:21.

As we near the close of time, we must rise higher and still higher upon the question of health reform and Christian temperance, presenting it in a more positive and decided manner. *Counsels on Health*, 467.

Still greater truths are unfolding for this people as we draw near the close of time, and God designs that we shall everywhere establish institutions where those who are in darkness in regard to the needs of the human organism may be educated, that they in their turn may lead others into the light of health reform. *Medical Ministry*, 187.

During the night we were in a council meeting, trying to decide what we were going to do. One of authority stood up and said, "Everything that has been given to ministers, to men in responsible positions, to teachers, to managers, to the different conferences, is to be repeated and repeated, because Satan is now doing a special work to make of no effect the testimonies that come from God. We must work earnestly to bring this instruction before the people." *Battle Creek Letters*, 3.

Regarding the testimonies, nothing is ignored; nothing is cast aside but time and place must be considered. Nothing must be done untimely. Some matters must be withheld because some persons would make an improper use of the light given. Every jot and tittle is essential and must appear at an opportune time. *Selected Messages*, book 1, 57.

Not one of the words which God has spoken must be allowed to fall to the ground. *Testimonies for the Church*, vol. 4, 517.

We know that in the past the truth has been demonstrated by the Holy Spirit. Not one word of human devising is to be permitted to subvert minds or to add unto or to take from the message that God has given. *The Paulson Collection of Ellen G. White Letters*, 200.

Time and trial have not made void the instruction given, but through years of suffering and self-sacrifice have established the truth of the testimony given. The instruction that was given in the early days of the message is to be held as safe instruction to follow in these, its closing days. *Review and Herald*, vol. 5, 342.

Abundant light has been given to our people in these last days. Whether or not my life is spared, my writings will constantly speak, and their work will go forward as long as time shall last. *Selected Messages*, book 1, 55.

Instructions Not Outdated by Science

WE ARE in the midst of a scientific revolution. New truths are being discovered nearly every day which require the modification or discarding of previously held "truths." Knowledge in some fields has been almost completely replaced within the last few decades. The principles of our health message are not susceptible to this scientific revolution. True science may help to round it out and confirm our message of health reform, but it will never replace it. Over one hundred years of intensive progress in science has only tended to confirm the principles of physiology, mental hygiene, environmental health, cause of disease, health preservation, and the treatment of disease as divinely revealed to us in the Bible and the Spirit of Prophecy. We tend to guard well this information. When some scientist, after years of intensive and costly research, shows that divine revelation has been correct all along, we too often re-read our counsel, smile smugly, and continue on our way. Scientists may never prove all of the counsel revealed to us, but this fact will never excuse us from acting upon it. Scientists tend to use in their approach to disease only those agents and methods which have been tested and proven effective.

HOWEVER, God expects His chosen people to accept and utilize in His health plan agents and methods which have not fully been proved by science. Righteousness (right doing) has always been by faith. The principles of right living given to us by God are to be accepted, practiced, and promulgated by faith. An eternity more of research cannot disprove them or replace them. God is the Author of our message of health as well as the Author of true science. One fears to wonder how many years and millions of dollars in research could have been spared by a greater faith in the origin of our message. One fears to wonder how much suffering and pain could have been prevented by a fuller acceptance of God's approach to disease. The past must not be the standard for the future. Let us go forward in faith.

Our Obligation

GOD HAS entrusted His work on earth to human beings. The success of His health program depends upon His people.

The divine strategy pays off only when we, in single-minded devotion, allow ourselves to become true instruments of God's plan. Editorial in *Scope*, July–August, 1972.

WHAT WILL be the spirit and motivation of those who carry God's program through to success?

The spiritual energies of His people have long been torpid, but there is to be a resurrection from apparent death. *Testimonies for the Church*, vol. 8, 297.

He who is truly converted will be so filled with the love of God that he will long to impart to others the joy that he himself possesses. Ibid., vol. 9, 30.

Just as surely as we receive, so surely must we give. None who receive the grace of Christ can keep it to themselves. As soon as Christ becomes an abiding presence in the heart, we shall not be able to see souls perishing in ignorance of the truth and be at rest. We shall make any sacrifice that we may reach them. *Medical Ministry*, 334.

He whose heart God touches is filled with a great love for those who have never heard the truth. Their condition impresses him with a sense of personal woe. Taking his life in his hand, he hurries away, a God-sent, God-inspired messenger, to do a work in which angels can cooperate. Manuscript,

73, 1901, *Health Education in the Seventh-day Adventist Church*, 223.

THE HOUR is late, the world's need is great. As God's called-out people with a Heaven-sent plan for the world's needs, we have a solemn obligation, a sacred commission.

Everywhere there are hearts crying out for something which they have not. They long for a power that will give them mastery over sin, a power that will deliver them from the bondage of evil, a power that will give health and life and peace. . . . The world needs today what it needed nineteen hundred years ago—a revelation of Christ. A great work of reform is demanded, and it is only through the grace of Christ that the work of restoration, physical, mental, and spiritual, can be accomplished. *The Ministry of Healing*, 142–143.

The world is in sad need of instruction along these lines. The time has come when each soul must be staunch and true to every ray of light God has given, and begin in earnest to give this gospel of health to the people. We shall have strength and power to do this, if we practice these truths in our own lives. If we all followed the light we have received, the blessing of God would rest on us, and we should be anxious to place these truths before those who know not. *Counsels on Health*, 446.

"Why," says one, "how can we do all this if the Lord is coming so soon?" Why, the Lord can do more in one hour than we can do in a whole lifetime, and when He sees that His people are fully consecrated, let me tell you, a great work will be done in a short time and the message of truth is to be carried into the dark places of the earth, where it has never been proclaimed. *Manuscript Releases*, Volume Five, 347.

Success Assured

GOD'S CALLED-OUT people have been trying to carry their message to the world for more than one hundred years. At this rate of progress one might question the possibility of success in our appointed work. When the progress to date is put along side of the immensity of the task, one can easily become disheartened and become negative in attitude. However, God's methods may be postponed through neglect or improper interpretation, but they can never be robbed of final victory. Heaven's Health Service is an integral part of God's final message to this earth, and it is predestined to succeed. The Lord Himself is confident of success. His attitude is positive and assuring.

> I will instruct the ignorant, and anoint with heavenly eyesalve the eyes of many who are now in spiritual darkness. I will raise up agents who will carry out My will to prepare a people to stand before Me in the time of the end. In many places that before this ought to have been provided with sanitariums and schools, I will establish My institutions, and these institutions will become educational centers for the training of workers. *Testimonies for the Church*, vol. 7, 101–102.

HEALTH reform will fulfill the purpose of its divine revelation.

> The Lord has presented before me that many, many will be rescued from physical, mental, and moral degeneracy through the practical influence of health reform. Health talks will be given, publications will be multiplied. The principles of health reform will be received with favor; and many will be enlightened. The influences that are associated with health reform will commend it to the judgment of all who want light; and they will advance step by step to receive the special truths for this time. *Medical Ministry*, 271.

MEDICAL Missionary work—a union of physical and spiritual healthcare—will be wholly successful.

> We shall see the medical missionary work broadening and deepening at every point of its progress, because of the inflowing of hundreds and thousands of streams, until the whole earth is covered as the waters cover the sea. *Medical Ministry*, 317.

> There will be a series of events revealing that God is master of the situation. The truth will be proclaimed in clear, unmistakable language. As a people we must prepare the way of the Lord

under the overruling guidance of the Holy Spirit. The gospel is to be given in its purity. The stream of living water is to deepen and widen in its course. In all fields, nigh and afar off, men will be called from the plow and from the more common commercial business vocations that largely occupy the mind, and will be educated in connection with men of experience. As they learn to labor effectively they will proclaim the truth with power. Through most wonderful workings of divine providence, mountains of difficulty will be removed and cast into the sea. The message that means so much to the dwellers upon the earth will be heard and understood. Men will know what is truth. Onward and still onward the work will advance until the whole earth shall have been warned, and then shall the end come. *Testimonies for the Church*, vol. 9, 96.

HEAVEN'S approach to the problem of disease is referred to as the right arm of the message. At times it appears to be a withered right arm, but it will not always be.

> Behold, the Lord's hand is not shortened, that it cannot save. Isaiah 59:1.

SUCCESS will require a supreme effort upon the part of every person. It will require complete faith in, and entire surrender and dedication to, God's plan. At times, discouragement may be overwhelming, but success is assured.

> There is no need to doubt or to be fearful that the work will not succeed. God is at the head of the work, and He will set everything in order. *Selected Messages*, book 2, 390. There is to be a working of our cities as they never have been worked. That which should have been done twenty, yes, more than twenty years ago, is now to be done speedily. The work will be more difficult to do now than it would have been years ago; but it will be done. *The Paulson Collection of Ellen G. White Letters*, 201.

> Fearful perils are before those who bear responsibilities in the Lord's work,—perils the thought of which makes me tremble. But the Word comes, "My hand is on the wheel, and in my providence I will carry out the divine plan." *Selected Messages*, book 2, 391.

THE EARTH groans under the weight of sin. Man's body, designed to last an eternity, barely ekes out an existence for seventy years before succumbing to the inroads of disease and misuse. But there is hope. God has given to His followers the Creator's Maintenance and Repair Manual for the human race. Let us not be disheartened. There is a way out. Our primary concern must be in regard to our relationship to Heaven's plan.

THE WORLD is in the midst of a health crisis. Humanly speaking, there can be no enduring solutions. God, however, has not been caught unprepared. There is a Heaven's Health Service and it is destined to revolutionize healthcare. Its success will be complete.

> And God shall wipe away all tears from their eyes; and there shall be no more death, neither sorrow, nor crying, neither shall there be any more pain; for the former things are passed away. Revelation 21:4.

LET IT be said that "There is balm in Gilead."

LET IT be said that "There is a prophet in Israel."

LET IT be said that "His people will respond in the day of His power."

LET IT be said that "There is a Heaven's Health Service."

A REFORMATION in healthcare is in progress. Let us ask ourselves the question "Will I, my family and my neighbors be participants in it?"

———————

www.ingramcontent.com/pod-product-compliance
Lightning Source LLC
Chambersburg PA
CBHW060002300526
45794CB00003B/1055